Banana Blossoms:
Banana Flowers

Banana Blossoms: Banana Flowers

Banana Blossoms: Banana Flowers

J. Z. PARKER

Banana Blossoms: Banana Flowers

J. Z. Parker, Copyright © 2024

ISBN: 9798882645839

Banana Blossoms: Banana Flowers

Contents

Banana Blossoms: Banana Flowers

About the Author

J. Parker believes that each choice you make regarding your food lifestyle acts as either a deposit into or withdrawal from your "health banking" account. You can choose to make mostly savings deposits or check withdrawals. The balance of that account determines your energy, vitality, risk of disease, longevity, and ultimately the quality of your life.

J. Parker has worked in big food companies creating concepts. J.Z. is also a pseudonym. J. Parker, fondly referred to as J.P., writes to inspire a healthy relationship with food and exercise, along with practical tips to incorporate healthy living.

Banana Blossoms: Banana Flowers

Chapter One: Introduction

Many parts of the banana tree are important. When we think of this tree all that comes to mind is the sweet banana we eat on daily basis. Even the banana leaves are important because in various parts of the tropics, the leaves are used as wraps for special slow cooking foods as they are steamed in the pots. Food such as tamales (Mexico), agidi and moi-moi (Nigeria) and pastel en hoja (Dominican Republic and Puerto Rico). Pasteles, also known as pastelles in the English-speaking Caribbean, are a traditional dish in several Latin American and Caribbean countries. In Puerto

Rico, the Dominican Republic, Trinidad and Tobago, the Caribbean coast of Colombia, and Panama plantain or banana leaves are used for wraps.

However the most ignored part of the banana tree can reverse aging, diabetes and polycystic ovary syndrome (PCOS). Like farmers, many house owners plant plantain and banana trees in their backyards and the trees will keep replicating itself for a very long period of time. The banana tree is a tree that keeps giving.

Banana flowers (a.k.a. banana blossoms) are, as the name suggests, the blossoms from a banana tree. At tail end of the bananas dangles the blossom. Like bananas, they are wonderfully edible. A picture of a banana tree is below.

There have been many studies on the benefits of banana blossoms. A study published in 2010 in "Journal of Chemical and Pharmaceutical Research" explains that banana flowers can help the process of wound healing and prevent infection.

Another study published in 2011 in

the journal "Research Parasitology" found that ethyl acetate extracts present in banana blossoms were able to inhibit the growth of "malarial parasite Plasmodium falciparum in vitro." Lots of banana blossom are consumed in India. India happens to be the largest cultivator of banana trees.

In India, banana blossoms can come in powdered form. Thankfully, some retail outlets in the West now carry the powdered form.

While India is probably the leading country in banana cultivation, the nutritional properties and health benefits of banana blossom are less researched. If people knew that the benefits can be altering—for the better—banana blossom would be a necessity to be had on a daily basis. Perhaps, new ways would be considered to process it more efficiently and its consumption increased.

The tedious preparation procedure for a dry or powdered banana blossom is perhaps reason why its price is exorbitant.

Considering all the benefits—which we will discuss in detail soon—factors in, the nutritional composition and antioxidant properties. The antioxidant properties is the catalyst that reverses and slows aging.

The fresh banana blossoms are the tender white hearts of the unopened, red tear-shaped banana flowers. Banana blossoms are a part of Indian, Thai, Vietnamese and Filipino cuisines. They are vegetables and are used in salad preparation. They can also be eaten raw, cooked in soups and stews. It can be fried also. Nature is a doctor. Nature has provided us with so many plants to meet our health needs. We just have to discover these medicinal plants.

The banana flower is a big, dark red blossom that grows from the end of a bunch of bananas. Some say the color is purple red. Purple buds appear from the heart of the tip of the stem and develop into tubular, milky colored flowers. The flavor has a little bitter taste. When cooked in a stew or soup, it is normally eaten as a complement to a dish. It is also a condiment in a salad.

Eating yellow bananas does the body good. It is good for your health but eating banana blossoms is even better. Though not widely eaten in the temperate regions, the banana flower is considered to be a vegetable in many parts of the world—

tropical areas—where the banana trees are cultivated.

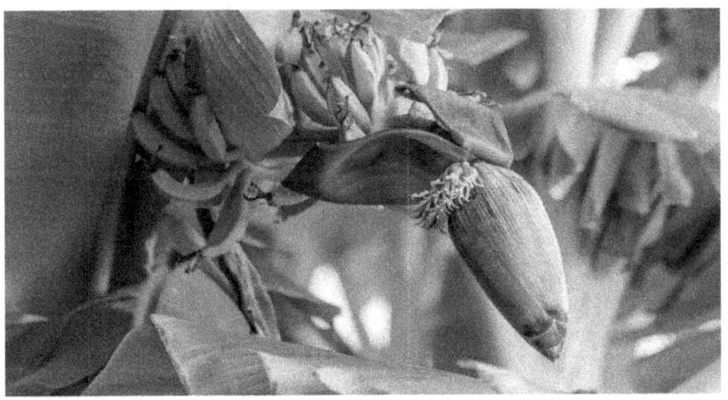

Picture of a Banana Tree, leaves and flower

The leaves from banana trees serve as food for some domestic animals like goats. Note that banana flowers are different from banana leaves. Banana leaves are heartier and thus more widely available. They are thick—even waxy—and a deep dark green. Banana leaves are not so much edible. They are used in many cuisines to wrap food for slow cooking. They do such with many Asian, African and Central American cuisines. They use them to wrap tamales (Mexico), Matoke (Uganda, Tanzania), Moi-Moi (Nigeria), for steaming in a pot. Banana leaves are widely used, up to this day for cooking and serving food in Africa, Asia and South America where they are available. I hope someday, some serious research will be done on banana leaves so that we can find how foods wrapped with banana leaves and cooked slowly last longer without spoiling.

Banana wraps served the purpose of modern-day refrigeration in that it kept food fresh for longer times. There is another purpose banana leave served. It prevents food from getting burnt and helps keep the heat in the food longer. You must have figured that properties (juices) in the banana leaves must have seeped unto the foods they were wrapped in before being slowly cooked. Therefore, the banana leave lends an aromatic and sweetish flavor to the cooked dish. Banana leaves serve as plates even to this day.

In some cultures around the globe, banana leave is "plate"

with which deities are served. Sometimes, we think our forefathers did not know much. They knew much more than we give them credit. Banana leaves contain natural antioxidants that get absorbed into the food during cooking. As an aside, if you are presented with choices of various foods—some wrapped in various leaves, others in fancy gold-plaited wares, you'd be very smart to choose those in wrapped natural leaves. You see, there is a reason to understand some of the practices of our past. There may be reason why our forefathers did it like that.

In some parts of India, banana leaves are used to serve food during festive and especially wedding meals. In some Asian countries, traditional foods are served on banana leaves even if supported with plates. That is—the plates are lined with banana leaves. Even here in our backyard, Americans in Puerto Rico, the dishes called arepas and sweet cassava tortilla are stored in banana leave wraps for a period before cooking. You can buy banana leaves and have it delivered the next day.

Let us leave banana leaves for now.

Where to Buy Banana Blossoms

1. Target
2. eBay
3. Walmart
4. Asian Grocery Stores
5. Etsy
6. Bonanza
7. Ypfarms (online)
8. Templeofthai (online)

Product can come fresh, frozen or canned (in brine).

Of course, fresh is best if you live in the tropics. You can go to your backyard and cut one whenever the need arises.

Tips for Using Banana Flowers

The darker, tough husks (often magenta in hue) on the outside of the flower need to be stripped away to reveal the tender, yummy yellow-green leaves inside. Banana blossoms will change color from yellowish gold to brown or black if left to sit and exposed to air for any length of time. It's like when you cut an apple in half and leave exposed for certain amount of time, it changes its color. In other words don't peel off that outer purple or reddish layer until you are ready to use them.

One way to minimize browning or blackening if there's a need to sit or expose the blossoms after you remove the tough outer layer, then separate the inner yellow and tender leaves, put them in a bowl of acidulated water. You can achieve this by adding several tablespoons of lemon juice to a bowl of water. You may also use vinegar. Add 1 tablespoon for every 2 cups of water to minimize the color change.

If your blossoms came in brine, you are set to go. Brine means water saturated or strongly impregnated with common salt. That is a way to keep the blossoms fresh. Read the directions on the container.

Perhaps you want the powdered (flour) type.

Chapter Two: How to Cook with Banana Blossoms

The enormous reddish or purplish-blue flower which comes from the banana plant is deliciously edible in salads, soups and stews. The thought of boiled yams or potato dipped in red thick stew full of banana blossoms and fish will make you salivate. In many banana producing countries, particularly those of South America, South East Asia and Africa, the curiosity of tourists is often aroused by recipes featuring what may at first sight, look like a huge artichoke, cooked in the same way as a vegetable. Also known as "banana heart", the inflorescence produced by this tropical plant will develop into a cluster of bananas. Banana blossom is often compared to artichokes. The taste too is similar—with a slight hint of bitterness. Banana blossom is also prepared like you would artichokes.

Preparation:

The external "petals", which are tougher and darker, have to be removed – but the fleshier ones can be stripped of their pulp. Then, one by one, the crisp leaves are peeled off to reveal the light-colored tender heart, the most prized part of the blossom. Cut into fine strips, the heart can be eaten raw in salads with a hot spicy sauce, as in the Thai dish nam prik or the Indonesian sambal – also excellent when teamed up with prawns and macadamia nuts. Like those of the artichoke, the petal-like leaves of the banana blossom will quickly oxidize on coming into contact with the air once cut because of their iron content, they will turn brown. It is advisable to dip them in acidulated water.

Cooking Banana Flowers:

Banana flowers is good for the preparation of crudités. Banana blossom can be cooked and used, for instance, to make delicious savory blossom fritters, which are popular in South India, Indonesia and Sri Lanka. It can be boiled in soups, possibly together with chicken and coconut milk. It may also be pan-tossed. Another popular cooking method is that of stewing. In the Philippines, for example, it is added to a type of stew—kari-kari. Kari-kari is the famous, tasty beef stew. If you happen to be a visitor in Philippines or Indonesia, you may wish to try out the kari-

kari or the pork sambal dishes respectively. There are other banana flower dishes sample.

In countries such as Laos and Thailand banana blossom dish is a staple. They are specialists when it comes to banana blossom dishes. Blossom is often used in combination with galangal root—a rhizome similar to its close relative, ginger. You can also coat the banana blossoms in the flour mixture. Then dip them in the batter. Gently lower the banana blossoms in the oil. Let them fry for about 4-5 minutes until golden brown, flipping them once.

Another preparation method: Step-by-step.

The ingredients

1 banana blossom, 1 lemon (squeeze to

remove seeds), water in a fairly large bowl

Preparation

a. Add the squeezed lemon juice
b. Remove the red petal about 3 to 4 layers into the banana blossom
c. Cut the banana blossom in half lengthwise
d. Core each blossom half
e. Thinly slice each blossom in half.

Immediately dip in the acidulated water to prevent browning

f. Do the same to the other cut half

g.   Let the banana blossom soak for about 5-6 hours. Some variety of blossom need to soak overnight. Note: You may wish to soak all varieties overnight.

h.   Drain out the acidulated water before eating, frying or cooking. Cook/fry no more than 4-5 minutes.

See picture below.

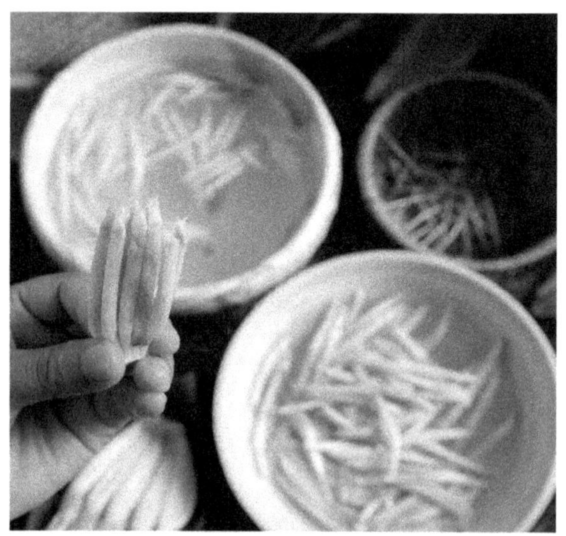

Banana Blossom Vegan Fish

A vegan fish made with banana blossom can be a delight. It is not only tasty but also very healthy. Using banana blossom in your dishes is like preventive cure to diabetes, bad cholesterol and those things that lead to bad health. A vegan fish with blossom as its base could be refreshing especially if you crave the taste for a fish. The soft yet crunchy and flaky texture of the banana blossom serves well for the fish base.

You can find a couple of "fishy" recipes with banana blossoms in vegan cookbooks. For preparation, follow the process for making tofish (fish made with tofu). Toss the banana blossoms in a flour mixture, then dip in a batter and fry until golden brown. Serve with baked potato or boiled yam or whatever you crave—with tartar sauce.

The *New York Times* ran a story aptly titled "In London's Vegan Fish-and-Chip Shop, Banana Blossoms Play Cod." It was a story about a vegan fish and chip shop but there is no fish involved in the menu served at Hackney's Sutton and Sons, and the fishless fish is made from banana blossoms. This tender flower has been a culinary staple in many Asian countries. It's "fish" from a banana tree that does not however taste anything like banana.

Banana leaves is served to domesticated animals. Banana leaves are tough and fibrous while banana blossoms are soft and tender. Banana blossom can be crunchy especially when deep fried. Some compare the taste to an artichoke when it comes to flavor. When sliced finely, fresh or canned banana blossom makes for a good addition to salads, and pairs well with many other foods. There is a Thai dish, a salad of banana blossoms, fried shallots, roasted chiles and a spicy rotisserie chicken is best paired with a few slices of roti.

Chapter Three: The Benefits of Banana Blossoms

We all know that vegetables are a must-eat food. Do you want to live healthily? If your answer is yes, then, vegetables and fruits must be a part of your diet. Among the various kinds of vegetables that are known, there is one that we don't seem to know about. This vegetable with its many benefits is cheap and is often left unused and untouched. It is the banana flower/blossom that is often served as a healthy diet. This vegetable gives your health a boost and a process of invigoration can be put in place, if you continuously eat dishes rich in banana blossoms. Let us read some of the benefits.

Prevents aging

Who wouldn't want to live a long and healthy life? Senescence is the gradual deterioration of the body due to age. The word senescence can refer either to cellular senescence or to senescence of the whole organism. Banana blossoms have the properties to actually delay or slow down the speed of this process—senescence. The amount of flavonoids in banana blossom, works to repair damaged body cells. It works as an antioxidant that prevents free radical attacks. Banana flowers are rich in vitamin C. It has compounds such as tannins and flavonoids. All of which are antioxidants. Antioxidant compounds help you to relieve stress conditions in our body's cells. Banana blossom works to slow the aging process. Banana blossom helps the prevention of the onset of premature aging problems.

Irregular Menstruation—

Banana flowers will help to overcome irregular menstruation. Eat lots of it, if you are experiencing such problems. The banana flower does this function by controlling the hormones in the body. It will therefore regularize your hormones and so, your period.

Reduces Menstrual Bleeding—The consumption of this vegetable is useful in overcoming bleeding problems during menstruation. This is because banana blossom can increase the level of progesterone in the body. Progesterone is used to cause periods in women who have not reached menopause but are not having periods due to a lack of this steroid in the body. Banana blossoms prevents excessive bleeding and is believed to overcome PCOS—polycystic ovary syndrome.

Enhances the Health of the Uterus—Foods enhanced with banana blossoms contain

minerals like calcium, vitamin C, iron and copper. These minerals help to strengthen the uterine wall and help to prevent infection in the uterus.

Reduce and Overcome High Cholesterol

Banana blossoms are helpful food eaten to avoid the occurrence of high cholesterol problems. Banana blossoms have an important content such as fiber. It is also low in fat. Banana blossoms have such a high degree of healthy content, it works to bind bad cholesterol and fat.

Smooth Blood Cycle—This is so because banana blossoms have anticoagulant properties that can prevent the build-up of blood clots.

Prevent Mumps—

This is because banana flowers contain iodine. There is no particular medication for the mumps virus but treatment is focused on alleviating mumps symptoms until the infection runs its course. However, diets containing banana blossoms keep mumps away.

Treating Malaria—

Malaria can be fatal if untreated. Banana

blossoms extract was discovered to kill the parasites that ultimately lead to full blown malaria. This is important to know especially knowing that the places where banana trees grow is also the places infested with mosquito.

Boosts Immunity—

Banana blossoms have antioxidant properties that prevent free radicals. It helps cell control and tissue damage. Like banana fruit, it can also boost our immunity against infection. Banana blossoms are thought to inhibit the growth of cancer cells. Banana blossoms helps you to overcome nausea, treat dizziness, strengthens teeth and gums.

Improves Memory—
Eat banana blossoms for a better long-term memory.

Strengthens Bones to Avoid Osteoporosis—

Osteoporosis cause your bone to become weak and brittle. The bones become so brittle that any applied pressure like a fall or coughing may result in broken bones. Osteoporosis-related fractures most commonly occur in the spine, wrist or hip.

Weight Loss—Banana

blossoms contain a high amount of fiber.

Roughage makes the stomach full quicker and remain full longer. When the stomach stays full for a longer period of time, you eat less.

Obesity Problems—
There are many problems associated with obesity. They are too many to cover here but be rest assured that obesity problems can result in death. This vegetable will serve an obese

individual well if eaten regularly. If you are obese, you might want to read about the health risks of overweight and how to lose the weight. Banana blossoms will enhance your efforts.

Nourishment of The Heart— The warding off of free radicals which is a benefit you get by eating healthy foods. Foods whose ingredients included fruits and vegetables especially banana blossoms is decision in the right direction. Banana flowers have high HDL fat content. High-density lipoprotein (HDL) cholesterol, sometimes referred to as the "good" cholesterol because it works to remove other, more harmful forms of cholesterol from your blood. It is believed that the higher your HDL levels are, the better and healthier you would be. Remembered the five most common heart problems are 1. Coronary artery disease 2. Heart attack 3. Hypertension 4. Stroke and 5. Arrhythmia.

Prevent Brain Cancer—Brain cancer can cause death. It is indeed a killer. Prevent it. Remove bad toxins from the body. It is simple. Eat banana blossoms. If you cannot lay your hands on the fresh banana blossoms, you can order the powdered form. Health is wealth.

Prevent Breast Cancer—Breast cancer is a killer. Prevent it. Eat lots of banana blossoms.

Helps to Overcome Anemia—Banana blossoms have a high content of iron. Iron is needed in the production of red blood cells. If you are anemic, stable consumption of this vegetable will help. Red blood cell functions as the transporter of oxygen throughout your body's cells. Your body needs iron in abundance to enable your body's daily activities. Banana blossoms are very rich in iron that enhances the processes the red blood cells will undertake in your body.

Neurological Disorder Problems—People who eat banana blossoms have the benefit of prevention for diseases such as Alzheimer's and Parkinson's. Such diseases happened in the first place because of the impact of free radicals dangerous to our wellbeing. Since banana blossoms contain high amount of antioxidants it serves to keep off free radical attacks.

Helps to Overcome Premenstrual Syndrome (PMS) Troubles—Banana blossoms are very good for alleviating PMS because its contents can prevent the symptoms associated with PMS. An addition of or pairing of yogurts with banana blossom enhances the efficacy to prevent PMS.

Banana blossoms contains magnesium which helps to enhance good mood, reduce stress and depression.

Wards off Free Radical Attacks—

There is consistency in our descriptions so far, that banana blossoms contain ingredients high in antioxidants. This is why its potency and efficacy is so beneficial to warding off free radicals that would otherwise cause harm to the body. Free radicals can cause cancer, lead to neurological disorders that enhance rapid deterioration into Alzheimer's and Parkinson's. Prevent such damages by what you eat especially with foods abundant with vegetables like banana blossoms.

Eat Banana Blossoms to Prevent Infection and Inflammation—

Banana blossoms contain anti-inflammatory properties. It also contain anti-bacterial properties. Due to these properties—anti-inflammatory and anti-bacterial, banana flowers can overcome health problems like ulcer, fungal infections, arthritis, and other inflammatory problems and infections.

Stop Diabetes—

Anyone experiencing diabetes is always careful of what s/he eats; especially with consumption of bread, soda, pasta and other sweet sugar foods. Banana flowers tend to decrease insulin levels in diabetic persons when consumed on a regular basis. The keyword here is—regular. You already know that banana flowers have pretty high fiber content which in turn, helps to prevent the rise in blood sugar level.

Improving the Mood— Everyone is entitled to good health and happiness. But not all will have both. If you are not healthy, you may not be happy. If you find yourself feeling frustrated on a daily basis, perhaps, you need to check what you are doing and eating. Do you feel like a zombie, waking up each day to what you think is a repetitive cycle that seems never-ending?

Has the quality of your life decreased over time, resulting in a loss of energy, vitality, and enthusiasm for a happy life? It could all be in your mood. A bad mood is a recipe for trouble—health wise— in the foreseeable future. Eat banana blossoms on a regular basis.

Not only does a healthy diet help control your waistline, but smarter food choices like dishes containing banana blossoms may also help ward off symptoms of depression. The best nutritional plan to help the mood is likely to be a varied diet with plenty of fruits and vegetables and others but make banana blossoms a staple. The richness in magnesium content of banana blossom helps improve a mood naturally instead of relying on prescription drugs with the attending negative effects.

Constipation Issues—

Due to banana flower's high fiber content, it is able to smooth the digestive system, so the problems of constipation can be tackled. Banana flowers contain insoluble fiber that is supposed to reduce the risk of constipation. Due to high fiber content, one gets the added benefit of both soluble and insoluble fibers working to keep your intestine clean and helps to maintain normal acidity level—a very important function to preventing the risk of colon cancer in our body's digestive system.

Activating Important Hormones—Hormones are tricky. Maintaining a harmonious dance between varieties of hormones is even trickier. While one hormone can be very important for human health, that same hormone can become detrimental to the body if produced in a limited or excess level and at a wrong time. There are lots of hormones like vitamin D, dopamine, adrenaline, thyroid, serotonin, progesterone, estrogen, testosterone, and etcetera. When you eat banana blossom, it has the ability to make all the hormones dance harmoniously, so to speak.

Increase Appetite— While this super food is able to reduce your food indulgence, it can also make those who eat less than needed to eat to their optimum for enhanced performance. In other words, banana blossoms works to make you attain your optimum health.

Amount of Hemoglobin—

Hemoglobin (Hgb) in blood transports oxygen from the lungs to the rest of tissues in our body. There it releases the oxygen so that aerobic respiration can take place to provide energy to power the functions of the organism in a process called metabolism. A healthy individual has 12 to 20 grams of hemoglobin in every 100 ml of blood.

Iron in banana blossoms is beneficial to increasing the production of HB. With optimum production you no longer are exposed to diseases of HB deficiency that is likely to cause the body to become pale and weak because of insufficient oxygen in the body cells.

Accelerate Wound Healing Process—

Wound healing is the restoration to normalcy an injured skin tissue. One way to sustain a wound is through surgery. It is believed that healthy sleeping routine can help boost the wound healing process. Eating your vegetables, the same study found, that nutritional supplements, in addition to healthy amounts of sleep, boosted the immune response in wounded persons.

One vegetable suited to boost the healing process is the banana blossoms. Some persons may have health issues like diabetes or blood clotting disorder that may inhibit normal healing process. Regular diets packed with banana blossoms will help the healing process.

Proteins—There is a high protein content in banana blossoms. So, banana blossoms, therefore, play a role in cell formation and regeneration. Proteins are biomolecules/macrom olecules with one or more long chains of amino acid residues. They perform a lot of functions inside our bodies. They perform catalyzing metabolic reactions, DNA replication etcetera, and mostly transport molecules from one place to another.

Fat Content—The content of fat contained in banana flowers can boost the process of cell formation and cell wall thickening. The cell wall can be tough, flexible, and sometimes rigid. Banana blossoms has properties that provides the cell with both structural support and protection. Banana blossom diet is suitable for those of you who are thinking of fattening the body. Mind you, don't worry about the word fat.

This fat is the good kind—HDL.

More Calories for Body Energy—Our daily calorie need on average is 2000 calories for women and 2500 for men. This vegetable can add calories. Reminder: Food is not plentiful all over the Earth in the same quantity as in a few places. So, available sources of calories must be identified and utilized.

A banana blossom dish is able to add those needed calories the body uses to generate the daily energy needs. Banana flowers can meet the number of calories a human body must reach daily in the process of burning energy.

Daily calorie intake in the United States.....3770

Daily calorie intake in the UK 3440

Daily calorie intake in Argentina
.....3000
Daily calorie intake in Ireland
.....3540
Daily calorie intake in India
.....2300
Suggested average calorie intake (women)...2000
Suggested average calorie intake (Men).....2500

Chapter Four:
Conclusion

This work has comprehensively detailed the composition and antioxidant properties of banana blossoms. Banana blossom in powder form is a by-product of banana trees. The analysis of banana blossoms showed their considerable antioxidant properties and nutritional value.

Banana blossoms powder was believed to contain a significant nutritive complement based on their high fiber content. Due to their high nutritional and antioxidant properties, banana blossoms can be used as ingredient in diets in the form of dehydrated powder. Banana blossom flour (powder) can be easily incorporated into food formulations.

However, where available, the fresh vegetable should be prepped and eaten raw, in a salad, or cooked/fried and paired with other diets. The resultant benefits show the potential of banana blossoms when eaten alone or paired with other foods. It is a huge source of natural antioxidants, phenols and flavonoids. With all the above health benefits, why wait to consume this stuff or pair it with your foods? Eat to live. Do not eat to accelerate your demise. Let the banana blossoms be an avatar to your health.

Every once in a while we learn of a new plant that opens us to new knowledge. You don't have to imagine what banana blossoms can do for you. You now know.

If you have read up to this page, you obviously likes good health counsel. And you are better positioned live a long and healthy life as you follow good eating habits. So, here is more good health news on another work on the benefits of another tree that you may be interested in. It's an e-book titled *PALM TREE*

OF LIFE: All You Need to Know about Palm Fruit Oil.

Be healthy, be happy. Always!

Other Kindle books by this author are listed below.

1.

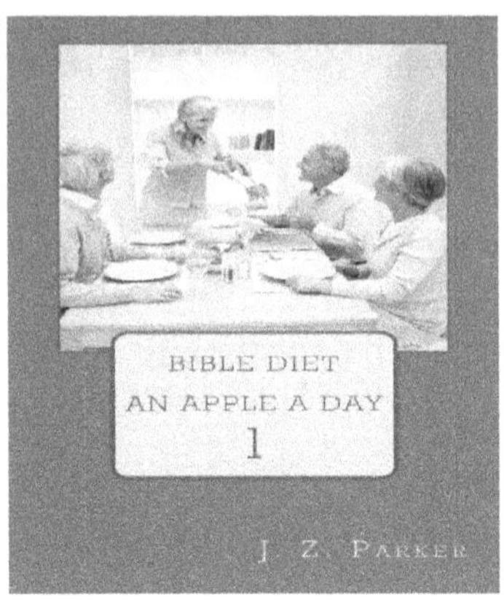

Gen 1:29 Then God said, "I give you every seed-bearing plant on the face of the whole earth and every tree that has fruit with seed in it. They will be yours for food. Gen 1:30 And to all the beasts of the earth and all the birds in the sky and all the creatures that move along the ground--everything that has the breath of life in it--I give every green plant for food." And it was so.

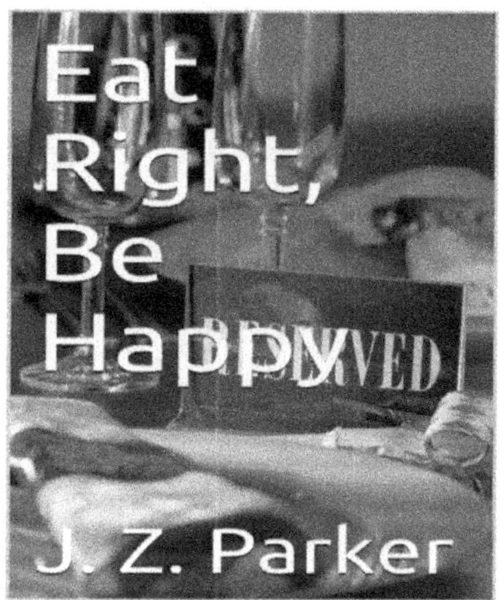

2.

Most often, being overweight is as a result of incapacitation. Overweight is a direct result of damaged communication between the body and the brain.

To some overweight individuals, the reward is in the food at all times from beginning to when the last piece of the food is eaten. Any more food brought immediately will still have the same reward.

3. Empower Your DNA: The Power of Vitamin C

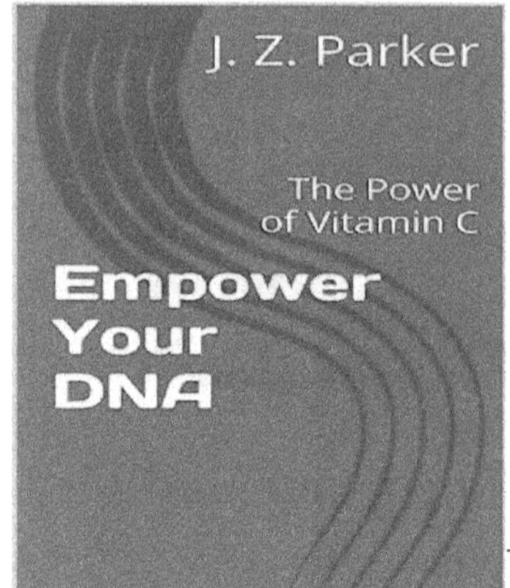

Many scientifically controlled studies using vitamin C for colds show that it can reduce the severity of cold symptoms, acting as a natural antihistamine. It can also be very useful for allergy control for the same reason: It reduces histamine levels. Because vitamin C gives your immune system one of the important nutrients it needs, extra vitamin C would often shorten the duration of the cold

Banana Blossoms: Banana Flowers as well.

4. Palm Tree of Life:

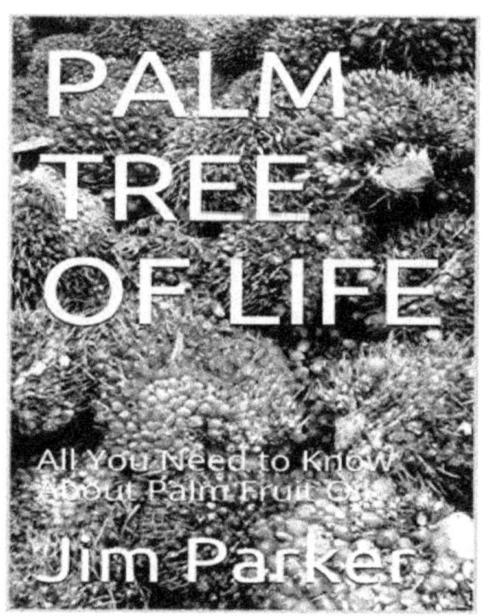

Nature has provided us with almost 600 known carotenoids, ranging from yellow orange to red hues and some of these possess Vitamin A activity of varying degrees. Palm fruit oil is one of the richest natural plant sources of carotenoids with concentration in the range of 500–700 parts per million—ppm.

5. Good & Bad Plastics: Bisphenol A:

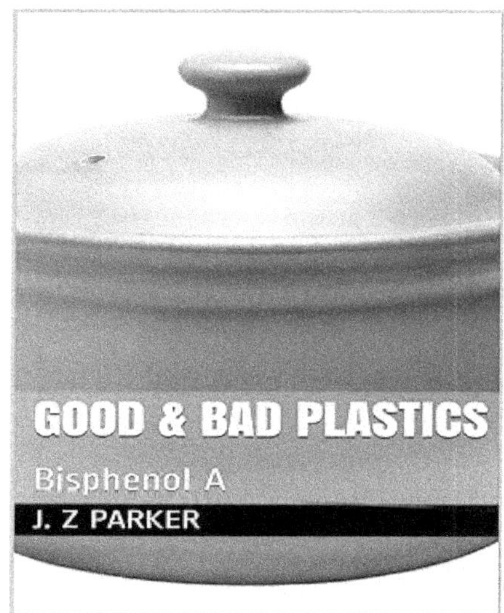

The wonder of canned food. Whip it open, heat it up in a plastic container and voilà, your meal is served. What is wrong with this picture? Did you notice the double whammy there? Some canned foods can affect your sex life negatively. They can also affect your libido negatively.

How is your food stored? If you buy canned foods—any can—then read on.

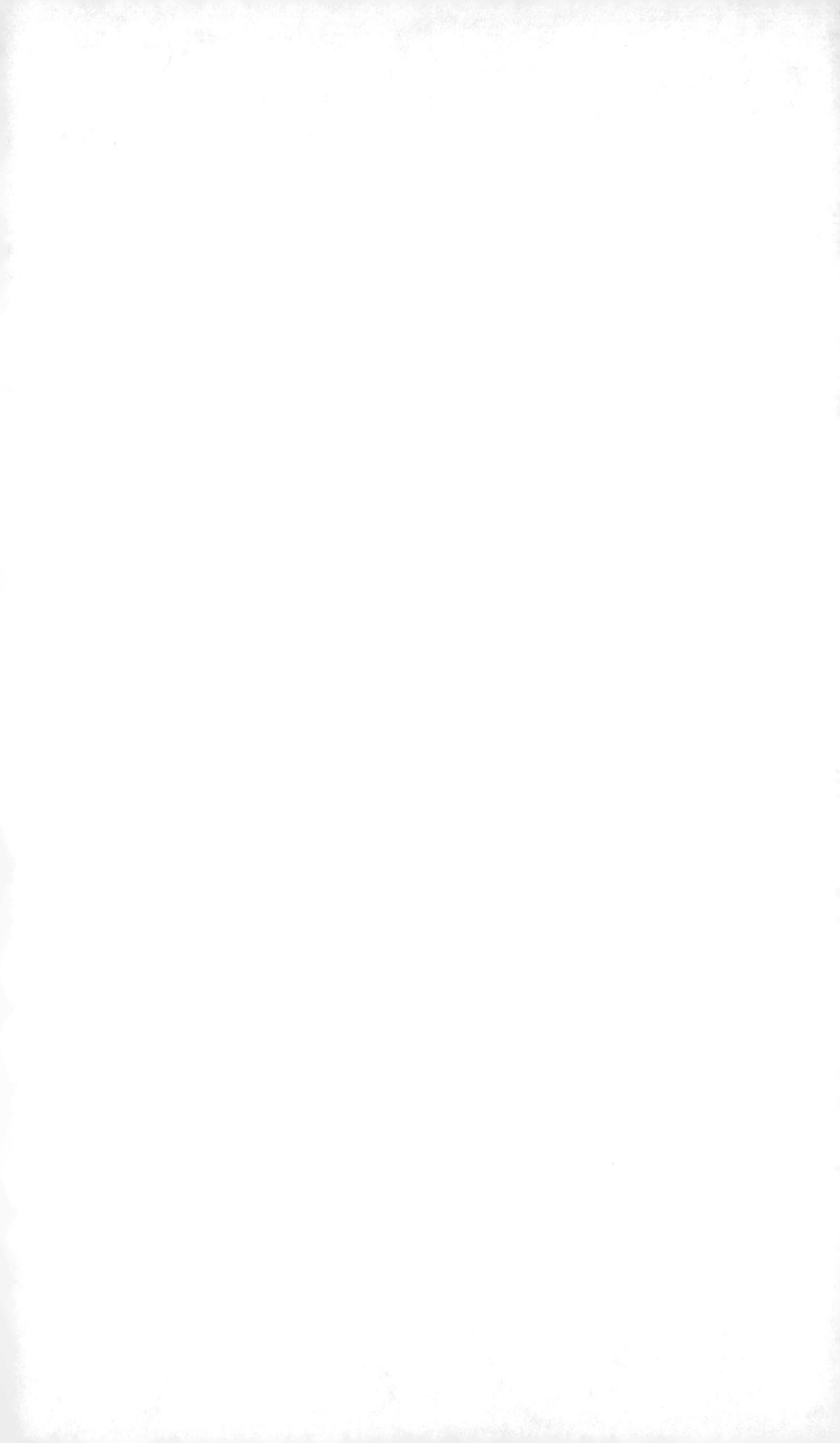

www.ingramcontent.com/pod-product-compliance
Lightning Source LLC
Chambersburg PA
CBHW070813280726

48660CB00015B/430